CARING FOR LOVED ONES WITH DEMENTIA

A PRACTICAL STRATEGIES AND EMOTIONAL SUPPORT BOOK

BY

DR SOFIA CARTER

Table of Contents

UNDERSTANDING DEMENTIA: TYPES SYMPTOMS AND PROGRESS 5

Types of Dementia...5

Symptoms and Progression 7

Conclusion 8

NAVIGATING THE EMOTIONAL IMPACT OF DEMENTIA CARE 9

Conclusion 11

CREATING A SUPPORTIVE AND SAFE ENVIRONMENT AT HOME 12

Conclusion 16

EFFECTIVE COMMUNICATION TECHNIQUES FOR DEMENTIA CARE 17

Conclusion 20

ESTABLISHING A STRUCTURED DAILY ROUTINE FOR STABILITY 21

The Benefits of a Structured Routine 23

Conclusion 26

MEMORY-STIMULATING ACTIVITIES AND COGNITIVE EXERCISES 27

The Importance of Memory-Stimulating Activities: 27

Conclusion 30

MANAGING CHALLENGING BEHAVIOURS WITH COMPASSION.............31

Conclusion 35

NUTRITIONAL CONSIDERATIONS FOR INDIVIDUALS WITH DEMENTIA ..37

Eating Challenges with Dementia 37

Suggestions for Easier Mealtimes..38

Nutrition Tips for Dementia Patients..40

Drinking Enough Fluids 42

Overeating 43

Feeding difficulties..46

Nutritional deficiencies..47

SEEKING EXTERNAL SUPPORT: RESPITE CARE AND COMMUNITY
RESOURCES..3...............48

Conclusion 51

FINAL CONCLUSION 52

INTRODUCTION

Caring for a loved one with dementia, a neurological condition characterized by a decline in cognitive function, including memory loss, impaired reasoning, and behavioural changes, presents a profound emotional and logistical journey for caregivers. Dementia, which often manifests in forms such as Alzheimer's disease, vascular dementia, and Lewy body dementia, affects not only the individual's cognitive abilities but also their emotional well-being and daily functioning. As the condition progresses, caregivers grapple with the challenges of providing compassionate care while loved ones. managing the evolving needs of their

Understanding the nuances of dementia's progressive nature, the unpredictability of symptoms, and the impact on both the individual and their support network is crucial for fostering an environment of empathy and effective caregiving. This guide is designed to offer caregivers comprehensive insights and practical strategies tailored to the different stages of

dementia. From establishing a structured daily routine that promotes familiarity and security to fostering open communication and implementing memory-stimulating activities, our aim is to provide a holistic approach that addresses the multifaceted demands of caring for individuals living with dementia. Furthermore, we emphasize the importance of self-care for caregivers, highlighting the significance of seeking emotional support and respite to sustain their well-being in this challenging yet profoundly meaningful caregiving journey.

CHAPTER ONE

UNDERSTANDING DEMENTIA: TYPES SYMPTOMS AND PROGRESS

Dementia, a broad term encompassing a range of neurological conditions, manifests as a progressive decline in cognitive function, impacting memory, reasoning, and behaviour. Understanding the complexities of dementia is crucial for caregivers as they navigate the multifaceted challenges of providing comprehensive care. This chapter provides an in-depth exploration of the different types of dementia, the associated symptoms, and the progressive nature of the condition.

Types of Dementia

- **Alzheimer's disease:** The most common form of dementia, Alzheimer's disease leads to memory loss, impaired judgment, and challenges with daily tasks. As the disease progresses, individuals may experience disorientation and difficulty communicating.

- **Vascular Dementia:** Caused by reduced blood flow to the brain, vascular dementia often results from stroke or other conditions affecting blood vessels. Symptoms may include difficulties with concentration, planning, and judgment, in addition to memory impairment.
- **Lewy Body Dementia:** Characterized by the presence of abnormal protein deposits in the brain, Lewy body dementia leads to fluctuations in alertness and attention, visual hallucinations, and symptoms similar to Parkinson's disease, such as tremors and rigidity.
- **Frontotemporal Dementia:** Affecting the frontal and temporal lobes of the brain, this form of dementia leads to changes in behaviour, personality, and language skills. Individuals may exhibit social and emotional disinhibition, apathy, or compulsive behaviour.

Symptoms and Progression

Early signs of dementia may include forgetfulness, difficulty finding words, and challenges with problem-solving. As the condition progresses, individuals may experience increased memory loss, confusion about time and place, and a decline in the ability to perform routine tasks. Changes in mood, behaviour, and personality may also become more pronounced, leading to heightened emotional challenges for both the individual and their caregivers.

Understanding the progressive nature of dementia is essential for caregivers to anticipate and address evolving care needs. Dementia often advances through stages, starting with mild cognitive impairment and progressing to moderate and severe stages characterized by significant memory loss and a decline in the ability to communicate and perform daily activities independently.

Conclusion

By comprehensively understanding the diverse types of dementia, the associated symptoms, and the progressive trajectory of the condition, caregivers can approach the caregiving journey with a heightened sense of awareness and preparedness. Recognizing the unique challenges posed by each subtype of dementia, caregivers can tailor their approach to meet the specific needs of their loved ones, fostering a compassionate and informed caregiving environment.

CHAPTER TWO

NAVIGATING THE EMOTIONAL IMPACT OF DEMENTIA CARE

Caring for individuals with dementia entails not only addressing their physical needs but also recognizing and managing the emotional toll that caregiving can have on both the caregiver and the individual, it is a journey that often elicits a wide spectrum of emotions. By fostering an understanding of the emotional dynamics at play, caregivers can create a compassionate and supportive environment that promotes the well-being of both themselves and their loved ones. As a caregiver, it is essential to recognize and navigate the emotional impact of providing care, ensuring that both the caregiver and the individual with dementia receive the necessary support and understanding. The following strategies can help in effectively managing the emotional aspects of dementia care:

- **Acknowledging Caregiver Stress and Burnout:** Providing care for someone with dementia can be emotionally demanding and physically exhausting. Acknowledge the signs of caregiver stress, such as feelings of isolation, irritability, or a sense of helplessness. It's crucial to prioritize self-care, seek respite, and access support systems to prevent burnout and maintain your well-being.

- **Cultivating Empathy and Patience:** Understanding the challenges faced by individuals with dementia can help cultivate empathy and patience in the caregiving process. Effective communication techniques, active listening, and responding with compassion can alleviate feelings of frustration and help in building a supportive environment that fosters a sense of security for the individual with dementia.
- **Addressing Grief and Loss:** Witnessing the gradual cognitive decline of a loved one can evoke a profound sense of grief and loss. It's essential to recognize and address these complex emotions. Acknowledge the

changes and losses experienced by both the individual with dementia and the caregiver, and seek support through counselling, support groups, or other resources to navigate the emotional journey with resilience and understanding.

Conclusion

By proactively managing the emotional impact of dementia care, caregivers can create a nurturing and compassionate environment that promotes the emotional well-being of both the caregiver and the individual with dementia. This approach fosters a deeper connection and understanding, enhancing the overall quality of life for everyone involved in the caregiving journey.

CHAPTER THREE

CREATING A SUPPORTIVE AND SAFE ENVIRONMENT AT HOME

Creating a supportive and safe environment at home is paramount in ensuring the well-being and comfort of individuals living with dementia. By implementing specific strategies and modifications, caregivers can promote independence, minimize potential hazards, and foster a sense of familiarity for their loved ones. The following approaches can be instrumental in establishing an environment conducive to the needs of individuals with dementia:

- **Assessing Home Safety:** Conduct a comprehensive assessment of the living space to identify potential safety risks and hazards. Ensure that the environment is well-lit, with clear pathways and minimal clutter to prevent accidents and promote ease of movement. Consider installing handrails, grab bars, and nonslip mats in areas prone to slips and falls, such as the bathroom and hallways.

- **Promoting Familiarity and Routine:** Maintain a consistent and predictable routine within the home environment. Create a structured daily schedule that incorporates familiar activities and tasks, as this can help reduce confusion and disorientation. Display familiar photographs, cherished mementos, and treasured possessions in prominent areas to evoke a sense of comfort and security for individuals with dementia.
- **Implementing Memory Aids and Reminders:** Integrate memory aids and reminders throughout the living space to support cognitive function and promote independence. Utilize labels on drawers and cabinets, place visual cues or signs to indicate the purpose of different rooms, and use calendars or whiteboards to display daily schedules and important appointments. These aids can help

individuals with dementia navigate their environment more confidently and maintain a sense of autonomy.

- **Minimizing Environmental Stressors:** Reduce environmental stressors that may cause agitation or confusion for individuals with dementia. Limit excessive noise, ensure a comfortable room temperature, and create a calming and soothing atmosphere by incorporating elements such as soft lighting, soothing colors, and familiar scents. This can help promote a sense of tranquillity and reduce feelings of anxiety or restlessness.
- **Ensuring Accessibility and Mobility:** Arrange furniture and household items in a way that promotes easy accessibility and encourages independence. Ensure that commonly used items are within reach, and consider using contrasting colors to distinguish essential objects and facilitate visual recognition. Make adaptations to the living space to accommodate any mobility aids, such as

walkers or wheelchairs, to promote safe and unhindered movement.

- **Encouraging Social Engagement:** Create opportunities for social interaction and engagement within the home environment. Arrange for visits from friends, family members, or community members, and foster meaningful social connections through activities such as storytelling, music listening, or simple group exercises. Facilitate a supportive and inclusive social environment that promotes a sense of belonging and emotional well-being for individuals with dementia.

- **Monitoring Changes and Adapting the Environment:** Continuously monitor changes in the individual's condition and adapt the home environment accordingly. Be responsive to evolving needs and preferences, and adjust the living space to accommodate any changes in cognitive abilities or physical capabilities. Regularly reassess the safety measures and environmental modifications to ensure that the living space remains conducive to the well-being and comfort of the individual with dementia.

Conclusion

By prioritizing safety, familiarity, and memory support within the home environment, caregivers can create a supportive and nurturing space that enhances the quality of life for individuals with dementia. These modifications not only foster a sense of security and comfort but also promote a greater sense of independence, a sense of connection, autonomy, and emotional well-being within the familiar surroundings of the home for those living with dementia.

CHAPTER FOUR

EFFECTIVE COMMUNICATION TECHNIQUES FOR DEMENTIA CARE

Effective communication plays a crucial role in establishing meaningful connections and fostering a supportive environment for individuals living with dementia. This chapter explores various communication strategies that can help caregivers navigate the unique challenges posed by cognitive changes, memory loss, and language difficulties. By employing these effective techniques, caregivers can promote understanding, reduce frustration, and enhance the overall quality of life for their loved ones.

- **Understanding Communication Challenges:** Communication challenges often accompany dementia, including difficulty finding words, impaired comprehension, and struggles with verbal expression. Caregivers must recognize and adapt to these challenges, remaining patient and attentive to the individual's needs.

Understanding the evolving communication abilities of individuals with dementia is essential in fostering clear and compassionate interactions.

- **Nonverbal Communication and Empathy:** Nonverbal communication, such as facial expressions, gestures, and tone of voice, can significantly enhance the emotional connection between caregivers and individuals with dementia. Caregivers should focus on conveying empathy and understanding through their nonverbal cues, fostering a sense of comfort and security for their loved ones. Maintaining eye contact, using a gentle touch, and employing a calm and reassuring tone can help establish a supportive and empathetic environment that encourages open communication and emotional connection.

- **Promoting Clear and Simple Communication:** Simplifying language and using clear, concise sentences can facilitate effective communication with individuals living with dementia. Avoiding complex explanations and using visual cues, such as gestures or props, can help convey messages more effectively. By promoting a straightforward and reassuring communication style, caregivers can reduce confusion and enhance understanding, fostering a sense of trust and comfort for individuals with dementia.

- **Encouraging Active Listening and Validation:** Active listening is a fundamental aspect of effective communication with individuals living with dementia. Caregivers should practice attentive listening, patience, and validation when engaging in conversations. Encouraging the individual to express their thoughts and feelings, even if they are fragmented or repetitive, can foster a sense of inclusion and self-worth. Validating their emotions and experiences by acknowledging their concerns and responding with empathy can help alleviate anxiety and promote a trusting and supportive relationship, enhancing the overall communication experience for both the caregiver and the individual with dementia.

Conclusion

By understanding the communication challenges associated with dementia and employing effective communication techniques, caregivers can establish a supportive and empathetic environment that promotes meaningful connections and emotional well-being. This chapter equips caregivers with the necessary tools and insights to navigate communication obstacles, fostering a positive and enriching caregiving experience for both the caregiver and the individual with dementia.

CHAPTER FIVE

ESTABLISHING A STRUCTURED DAILY ROUTINE FOR STABILITY

Maintaining a structured daily routine for individuals living with dementia is crucial for providing a sense of stability and security. By establishing a predictable schedule, caregivers can help reduce feelings of confusion and disorientation, which are common challenges faced by those with dementia. A structured routine provides a framework for the day, incorporating familiar activities and tasks that help individuals feel more at ease and in control of their environment.

One of the key benefits of a structured routine is that it can significantly minimize distress and agitation, as individuals with dementia often find comfort in familiarity and predictability. By establishing regular times for meals, activities, and rest, caregivers can create a sense of rhythm that fosters a more stable and reassuring atmosphere. Consistency in daily routines can also aid in regulating sleep patterns, contributing to improved overall well-being and a better quality of life for individuals with dementia.

In designing the daily routine, it is essential to consider the individual's preferences, interests, and abilities. By incorporating activities that the individual enjoys and finds meaningful, caregivers can promote engagement and a sense of purpose. These activities can include hobbies, pastimes, or simple tasks that resonate with the individual's personal history and experiences. By tailoring the routine to the individual's likes and dislikes, caregivers can encourage active participation and stimulate cognitive and emotional well-being.

While maintaining structure is important, it is equally vital to remain flexible and adaptable to accommodate changes in the individual's mood, energy levels, and cognitive abilities. Caregivers should be attuned to the individual's nonverbal cues and adjust the routine accordingly. Being responsive to the individual's needs fosters a supportive and nurturing environment that respects their autonomy and promotes a sense of well-being.

By establishing a structured daily routine that combines familiarity, tailored activities, and flexibility, caregivers can create an environment that enhances the overall quality of life for individuals living with dementia. This approach promotes a sense of stability, purpose, and comfort, contributing to a more enriching and fulfilling daily experience for both the caregiver and the individual receiving care.

The Benefits of a Structured Routine

- **Promoting a Sense of Security:** A structured routine provides a predictable and secure environment, reducing feelings of uncertainty and anxiety that individuals with dementia may experience. Consistent daily activities and schedules can foster a sense of stability and comfort, promoting a greater sense of security and well-being.
- **Enhancing Cognitive Functioning:** Following a structured routine can help stimulate

cognitive abilities and memory retention for individuals with dementia. Engaging in familiar activities at regular intervals can aid in maintaining cognitive function and preserving a sense of familiarity, contributing to the overall cognitive well-being of the individual.

- **Minimizing Behavioural Challenges:** By providing a clear and structured daily schedule, caregivers can help minimize disruptive behaviours often associated with dementia, such as agitation, restlessness, and aggression. A consistent routine can help reduce confusion and frustration, leading to a more calm and harmonious environment.

- **Facilitating Independence:** A structured routine that includes simple and familiar tasks encourages individuals with dementia to participate in daily activities independently. This can promote a sense of accomplishment and autonomy, boosting the individual's self-esteem and fostering a greater sense of independence and control over their environment.

- **Supporting Physical Well-being:** A well-structured routine ensures that individuals with dementia receive regular meals, physical activities, and adequate rest, thereby supporting their overall physical health. Regular exercise, proper nutrition, and sufficient rest contribute to improved physical well-being and can help minimize health-related complications associated with dementia.

- **Promoting Emotional Well-being:** Following a consistent and engaging routine can have a positive impact on the emotional well-being of individuals with dementia. Engaging in enjoyable activities and maintaining social connections through structured routines can promote feelings of happiness, contentment, and emotional fulfilment, fostering a more positive and enriching daily experience.

Conclusion

By embracing the concept of a structured daily routine, caregivers can provide a nurturing and enriching environment that not only supports the immediate needs of individuals with dementia but also contributes to their long-term emotional and physical well-being. This approach fosters a sense of purpose, autonomy, and dignity, enabling individuals with dementia to lead a more fulfilling and meaningful life within the comfort of their home environment. Furthermore, a structured routine serves as a cornerstone for maintaining a sense of normalcy and familiarity, even as the cognitive abilities of individuals with dementia may change over time. It offers a source of comfort and security, creating an environment that promotes emotional well-being and fosters a greater sense of connection and understanding between caregivers and their loved ones.

CHAPTER SIX

MEMORY-STIMULATING ACTIVITIES AND COGNITIVE EXERCISES

Engaging individuals with dementia in memory-stimulating activities and cognitive exercises is essential for maintaining cognitive function, promoting mental stimulation, and enhancing overall well-being. This chapter explores various techniques and activities that can help preserve memory, stimulate cognitive abilities, and foster a sense of accomplishment and enjoyment for individuals living with dementia.

The Importance of Memory-Stimulating Activities:

- Memory-stimulating activities play a crucial role in slowing cognitive decline and preserving memory function for individuals with dementia. By engaging in activities that encourage mental agility and stimulate memory recall, individuals can experience improved cognitive retention and a heightened sense of cognitive well-being. Such activities also promote a sense of accomplishment and self-esteem, contributing to a more positive and fulfilling daily experience.

- **Tailoring Activities to Individual Preferences:** Tailoring memory-stimulating activities to align with the individual's preferences, interests, and abilities is essential for promoting engagement and a sense of enjoyment. Caregivers should consider incorporating activities such as reminiscence therapy, puzzles, music therapy, and sensory stimulation, based on the individual's past experiences and personal interests. By providing activities that resonate with the individual's unique background, caregivers can create a meaningful and enriching experience that encourages active participation and promotes emotional well-being.

- **Incorporating Cognitive Exercises:** Cognitive exercises are instrumental in maintaining cognitive function and promoting mental acuity for individuals with dementia. These exercises may include simple tasks such as word games, problem-solving activities, and visual-spatial exercises that stimulate various cognitive domains. By incorporating a variety of cognitive exercises into the daily routine, caregivers can support the individual's cognitive abilities and enhance their overall cognitive well-being, leading to a more fulfilling and enriching quality of life.

- **Encouraging Social Interaction and Engagement:** Promoting social interaction and engagement within the context of memory-stimulating activities can foster a sense of connection and belonging for individuals with dementia. Group activities, social gatherings, and interactive games provide opportunities for individuals to engage with others, fostering a supportive and inclusive environment that promotes emotional well-being and a sense of community.

Conclusion

By incorporating memory-stimulating activities and cognitive exercises into the daily routine, caregivers can create a nurturing and enriching environment that supports the cognitive well-being and overall quality of life for individuals living with dementia. This chapter provides caregivers with practical insights and strategies to implement engaging and meaningful activities that stimulate memory, promote cognitive function, and foster a positive and fulfilling daily experience for their loved ones.

CHAPTER SEVEN

MANAGING CHALLENGING BEHAVIOURS WITH COMPASSION

Caring for individuals with dementia often involves addressing challenging behaviours that can arise as a result of the cognitive and behavioural changes associated with the condition. Managing these behaviours with compassion and understanding is essential in ensuring the well-being and comfort of both the individual and the caregiver and also an aspect of providing care for individuals living with dementia. These behaviours, often stemming from the complex interplay of cognitive decline, environmental stressors, and unmet needs, can pose significant challenges for both caregivers and individuals with dementia.

- **Recognizing Unmet Needs and Addressing Distress:** Understanding that challenging behaviours in individuals with dementia may stem from unmet needs or emotional distress is vital for providing compassionate care. Individuals with dementia may experience difficulty expressing their needs, leading to frustration and agitation. Caregivers can employ a keen observation of nonverbal cues and changes in behaviour to identify underlying discomfort or unmet needs, such as hunger, pain, or a need for social interaction. By addressing these needs promptly and empathetically, caregivers can alleviate distress and reduce the occurrence of challenging behaviours.

- **Implementing Person-Centered Care for Dementia Behaviours:** Adopting a person-centered approach tailored to the unique needs and preferences of individuals with dementia is essential in managing challenging behaviours with compassion. Creating a supportive and familiar environment that accommodates the individual's specific routines and interests can foster a sense of security and reduce feelings of distress. By prioritizing the individual's autonomy and dignity, caregivers can build a trusting relationship that promotes a more positive caregiving experience.

- **Promoting Effective Communication Strategies:** Utilizing effective communication strategies is key in managing challenging behaviours with compassion for individuals with dementia. Employing simple and clear language, using nonverbal cues, and maintaining a calm and reassuring tone can help prevent misunderstandings and minimize agitation. Encouraging active listening and validating the individual's feelings can foster a sense of emotional connection and understanding, reducing the likelihood of escalated behaviours.

- **Integrating Meaningful Activities and Routines:** Incorporating meaningful activities and consistent routines tailored to the individual's abilities and interests can provide a sense of purpose and engagement for individuals with dementia. Engaging in familiar tasks, hobbies, or reminiscence activities can help reduce boredom and restlessness, contributing to a more positive and fulfilling daily experience. By focusing on activities that evoke positive memories and emotions, caregivers can foster a sense of joy and emotional well-being.

- **Collaborating with Healthcare Professionals and Support Networks:** Collaborating with healthcare professionals and engaging with support networks can provide valuable guidance and assistance in managing challenging behaviours with compassion. Seeking advice from geriatric specialists, dementia care experts, and support groups can offer caregivers access to valuable resources, training, and emotional support. Consulting healthcare professionals for personalized care plans and medication management strategies can ensure a comprehensive and holistic approach to addressing challenging behaviours, promoting the overall well-being and quality of life for individuals with dementia.

Conclusion

By managing challenging behaviours with compassion in the context of dementia care, caregivers can create a nurturing and understanding environment that promotes the emotional well-being and dignity of individuals living with dementia. Managing challenging behaviours with compassion in the context of dementia care demands a multifaceted and empathetic approach that prioritizes the individual's emotional well-being and dignity. By recognizing the complex interplay of cognitive decline, unmet needs, and emotional distress, caregivers can respond with patience, empathy, and understanding, fostering a supportive and nurturing environment. Incorporating positive reinforcement, creating a calming physical space, and collaborating with healthcare professionals and support networks are essential components of a comprehensive and compassionate care approach. By implementing these strategies, caregivers can cultivate a more peaceful and enriching caregiving experience that promotes the overall quality of life and emotional comfort for individuals navigating the complexities of dementia.

CHAPTER EIGHT

NUTRITIONAL CONSIDERATIONS FOR INDIVIDUALS WITH DEMENTIA

Nourishment plays a vital role in supporting the overall health and well-being of individuals with dementia. The dietary needs of those living with dementia can significantly differ due to various factors, including changes in appetite, cognitive decline, and swallowing difficulties. By understanding the importance of a well-balanced diet and implementing strategies to overcome dietary obstacles, caregivers can contribute to the individual's physical health, cognitive function, and emotional well-being.

Eating Challenges with Dementia

- Weight loss is common and tends to become more severe as dementia gets worse.
- Food may taste bland due to changes in sense of smell and taste.

- Coordination skills might decline, making use of eating utensils or feeding oneself difficult.
- Chewing and swallowing problems can make it difficult to eat. Some prescribed diets include softer foods to help encourage intake or thickened liquids for easier swallowing.
- With severe dementia, individuals may also lose the ability to distinguish food from non-food objects.

Suggestions for Easier Mealtimes

Simplifying the act of eating and making it a more social activity can help a person with dementia stay engaged and well-nourished. Here are some tips which can make it easier for them to eat healthily and enjoy their mealtimes. Do note that while it is important you allow them to feed themselves, you should also be prepared to step in and help when necessary.

- **Avoid Distractions During Meals:** To keep your loved one from getting overwhelmed or confused during meals, eat in a calm and quiet environment together. While talking to each other is encouraged, turn off the television and radio to minimise distraction.

- **Enjoy Meals Together:** Make eating a more social activity that will help keep your loved one engaged, so they will continue to look forward to mealtimes.

- **Have Small, Healthy Snacks Available:** People with dementia may have trouble recalling that they had just eaten a meal, prompting them to ask when breakfast or dinner will be served. Instead of telling them that they just ate, offer them small healthy snacks. Raisins, dried fruit, and yoghurt are all healthy food that can satiate their cravings in a nutritious way.

- **Give Plenty of Time to Finish Meals:** Because of impaired coordination, dementia sufferers may take much longer to cut food, chew, and swallow. Be patient with your loved ones and expect mealtimes to be longer. Let them take their time to eat. This will help preserve a sense of normalcy and independence in a dementia patient.

- **Provide Finger Foods:** The easier it is for your loved one to eat, the more they can enjoy their mealtime and get all their nutrients. Give them bite-sized items such as steamed broccoli, orange segments, and chicken nuggets, which they can easily pick up and consume even without utensils.

Nutrition Tips for Dementia Patients

A healthy, balanced diet is vital for dementia individual. Enjoying foods from all the different food groups is important to provide the body with all the nutrients it needs.

Studies have shown that certain combinations of nutrients may help to support healthy brain function. Because dementia affects mobility and the senses, it is advisable to try and make every meal a healthy one. This minimises the negative impact of skipped meals or overeating and can help a person with dementia stay fit.

Here are some quick and easy tips for creating a nutritious meal plan.

- **Cut Down Refined Sugar Intake:** Refined sugar has lots of calories but no essential vitamins and minerals. Excessive sugar intake such as high consumption of added sugar beverages, added sugar desserts or overly sweet fruits has been linked to declines in memory, cognitive and other brain functions. If your loved one's dementia is giving them a sweet tooth, satisfy their sugar cravings with naturally sweet food such as fruit lightly sweetened smoothies.

- **Reduce Sodium Consumption:** Sodium can elevate blood pressure to dangerously high levels. High sodium diet has been identified as risk factor of hypertension and cardiovascular disease, both of which are linked to dementia. Reduce the salt intake for your loved one and flavour their food with fresh herbs and spices instead. It is also crucial to pay attention to hidden sources of sodium in pre-made meals and processed food and control intake of foods such as canned meat and fish, bacon, sausage, spam, salted nuts, frozen meal, etc.

- **Provide a Balanced, Varied Diet:** Ensure that their daily meals always have a healthy mix of lean proteins, whole grains, low-fat dairy items, fruits, and vegetables. Check out top food ideas to increase appetite and promote good nutrition in elderly adults from our blog article here.

Drinking Enough Fluids

Persons living with dementia who are older may be more susceptible to dehydration due to reasons such as a blunted sense of thirst, poor memory, immobility or medications interfering with their thirst mechanism. Low hydration levels are associated with incidences of acute confusion/delirium, urinary tract infections, constipation and delayed wound healing. Fluids include milk, tea and coffee, water, fruit juice, and other soft drinks and liquid foods. A total of approximately 6-8 cups (1.5 – 2 litres) of fluid a day is recommended unless otherwise specified by a doctor or specialist nurse. To help the person with dementia drink enough:

- Offer fluids frequently throughout the day in an appropriate cup. Gentle reminders and prompts to drink may help such as placing the hand on the cup. Offering the cup rather than leaving it on the table may prompt a person to drink.
- Consider carbonated drinks to stimulate the senses.
- Encourage the consumption of foods with a high fluid content e.g. jelly, soup, ice cream, yoghurts and sauces.
- Offer drinks after, instead of with the meal, or only offer small amounts during the meal and a full drink afterwards.

Overeating

Sometimes people with dementia may start to gain excessive weight or eat more than usual, or start asking for food even though they have just eaten a full meal. This can be distressing for people looking after them, and carers can feel uncomfortable telling someone that they have already eaten. Weight gain or eating extra portions should only be a concern if it is causing health-related problems, or if the person is uncomfortable or distressed. There are many reasons which may contribute to over-eating:

- Consider whether the person may be depressed or had a medication change which has impacted on their appetite or weight – ask their GP for a review
- Consider if the person is bored or lonely and is finding comfort in food – in this case, focus on helping them to manage these feelings other than eating

These tips will help you manage their eating habits

- Divide meals into two smaller portions and when food is requested the second time, give the second portion
- Serve a small portion of protein (fish, meat, poultry or vegetarian alternative) and starchy carbohydrate foods (potatoes, rice,

pasta or bread) and fill most of the plate with salad or vegetables
- Offer low calorie snacks such as fruit or light yoghurt as an alternative to an extra meal
- Make ice-lollies with sugar-free or diet drinks. Offer these as a snack or a second dessert.
- Provide lower-energy drinks such as tea or coffee, diet, sugar-free or reduced-sugar squash/fizzy drinks, or water
- Use sweeteners instead of sugar
- Use low fat dairy products like low fat cheese, and skimmed or semi skimmed milk
- Grill or oven cook foods instead of frying
- Encourage the person to be as active as they are able
- Try and determine whether the person is aware of the changes in their eating habits and how they feel about this. Food and drinks should never be taken away or hidden from a person who has the capacity to make choices about what they want to eat

Feeding difficulties

If the person finds sitting down for a long time is difficult, eating a plated meal can be challenging. Agitation burns extra energy and can contribute to weight loss. Consider:

- Changing the environment e.g. limit distractions by turning off the television or radio and provide background noise such as soothing music
- Whether there are times in the day when the person is more settled and then change mealtimes or offer additional snacks at these times
- Placing food in the person's hand to prompt them

People with dementia can get 'stuck' saying the same thing. If food is verbally refused, offer something again 15-30 minutes later. If food refusal continues, seek advice from a GP as this may indicate other issues

Nutritional deficiencies

Nutritional deficiencies can be common in the following:

- Folate-deficiency anaemia is common in people with dementia. Good examples of folate are fruits, vegetables, fortified breakfast cereals and yeast extract. Try and include these in your daily diet.
- Vitamin and mineral intake can be inadequate in people with dementia so a general multivitamin supplement may be beneficial, especially if dietary intake is very limited. A GP or Dietician can provide guidance on this.

Note: For people with a poor appetite and weight loss, high fibre foods can fill them up before they have eaten enough energy to meet their needs. In this case, lower fibre options may be better, or introduce higher fibre options in small portions and monitor.

CHAPTER NINE

SEEKING EXTERNAL SUPPORT: RESPITE CARE AND COMMUNITY RESOURCES

The journey of caregiving for individuals with dementia can present unique challenges that often necessitate external support in the form of respite care and community resources. This chapter sheds light on the critical role of seeking assistance from specialized care services and community-based programs tailored to the specific needs of individuals living with dementia. By understanding the value of these external support networks, caregivers can access practical assistance, emotional solace, and valuable resources that not only alleviate the burdens of caregiving but also enhance the overall well-being and quality of life for both the caregivers and the individuals in their care.

- **Exploring the Benefits of Respite Care for Dementia:** Recognizing the benefits of respite care is crucial for caregivers in need of temporary relief from the demanding responsibilities of dementia care. Exploring various respite care options, such as in-home care, adult day programs, and short-term residential facilities, can provide caregivers with the opportunity to recharge and tend to personal needs, knowing that their loved ones are receiving expert and compassionate care in a safe and supportive environment.

- **Engaging with Dementia-Specific Community Programs:** Active engagement with community programs tailored to the unique needs of individuals with dementia can foster a sense of belonging and emotional support for both the caregivers and the individuals in their care. Participating in memory enhancement workshops, support groups, and recreational therapy sessions can provide cognitive stimulation, social interaction, and emotional comfort, creating a nurturing community that understands and embraces the challenges of dementia caregiving.

- **Navigating Legal and Financial Resources:** Navigating the complex legal and financial aspects of dementia care is essential for caregivers in ensuring the long-term well-being and security of their loved ones. Understanding the intricacies of estate planning, insurance coverage, and government assistance programs can empower caregivers to make informed decisions and access the necessary resources to provide comprehensive and sustainable care for individuals with dementia.

- **Harnessing Technological Solutions for Dementia Care:** Harnessing the power of technology and digital resources can offer caregivers valuable tools and platforms for managing the multifaceted demands of dementia care. Leveraging telehealth services, remote monitoring tools, and online support networks can provide caregivers with accessible guidance, real-time assistance, and virtual connections, offering a more streamlined and efficient approach to addressing the diverse needs of individuals with dementia.

Conclusion

By proactively seeking external support through respite care and community resources, caregivers can access a network of assistance and guidance that not only alleviates the challenges of dementia care but also promotes their well-being and resilience. This chapter equips caregivers with practical insights and resources to explore specialized respite care options, engage with dementia-specific community programs, navigate legal and financial considerations, and harness technological solutions, fostering a more comprehensive and sustainable approach to dementia caregiving.

CHAPTER TEN

FINAL CONCLUSION

"Caring for Loved Ones with Dementia: Practical Strategies and Emotional Support" serves as a guiding light for those undertaking the challenging yet deeply rewarding journey of caring for individuals with dementia. By understanding the diverse aspects of dementia, including its types, symptoms, and progression, caregivers can develop a comprehensive approach that encompasses effective communication techniques, memory-stimulating activities, and structured daily routines.

Throughout this book, we have explored the significance of creating a supportive and safe environment at home, where individuals with dementia can find comfort and familiarity amidst their cognitive challenges. Navigating the emotional impact of dementia care has been emphasized, recognizing the essential role of empathy and compassion in fostering a nurturing and respectful caregiving environment.

Addressing the nutritional considerations specific to individuals with dementia has underscored the importance of tailored meal plans and hydration strategies that promote overall well-being and cognitive function. Additionally, the exploration of respite care and community resources has shed light on the significance of accessing external support networks that can offer practical assistance, emotional solace, and valuable resources for both the caregivers and their loved ones.

As we conclude this journey, let us remember that while caring for loved ones with dementia may present its share of challenges, it also offers moments of profound connection, joy, and shared experiences. By implementing the practical strategies outlined in this book and nurturing a culture of empathy and understanding, caregivers can create a supportive and enriching environment that promotes the dignity, well-being, and quality of life for individuals with dementia and let us embrace the profound lessons learned and the deep connections fostered throughout the process of caring for loved ones with dementia. May this resource serve as a beacon of hope, guidance, and empathy, empowering caregivers to navigate the complexities of dementia care with unwavering compassion, patience, and unwavering dedication.